THE ULCERATICE COLITIS COOKBOOK

Nutritious and Delicious Recipes for Managing Ulcerative Colitis

Antone Blick

COPYRIGHT

TABLE OF CONTENTS

INTRODUCTION

Ulcerative colitis (UC) is a chronic condition that causes inflammation of the large intestine (colon) and the rectum and sores (ulcers) on the inner lining of the large intestine. Ulcerative colitis is thought to be an autoimmune disease, that is, one where the body attacks itself. It is a type of inflammatory bowel disease (IBD). It is not the same as Crohn's disease, another type of IBD, which can affect any part of the gastrointestinal tract, whereas ulcerative colitis only affects the colon and rectum. It is also not the same as irritable bowel syndrome (IBS), which affects how the colon functions and does not cause inflammation.

Ulcerative colitis is estimated to affect nearly 907,000 Americans, and it affects males slightly more often than females. The disease is most commonly diagnosed between the ages of 15 and 40.

Many people who have ulcerative colitis or another form of IBD find a diet that works well for them and choose to remain on it even when they are not actively having symptoms (a period of remission), as it may help them keep flares at bay.

Research has indicated that many people who have mild-to-moderate ulcerative colitis benefit from making changes to their diet in conjunction with other treatments (such as medication).

Studies have also indicated that the quality of life for people with ulcerative colitis and other forms of IBD may be particularly influenced by their diet (what researchers refer to as "food-related quality of life").

If your digestive tract is inflamed because of a condition like ulcerative colitis, certain kinds of food and drink may worsen your symptoms. For instance, spicy foods or those that are high in fat (like fried foods) may trigger certain symptoms.

People who have severe ulcerative colitis may also experience certain complications, such as strictures, that require them to avoid entire food groups or adhere to a certain type of diet for a longer period of time.

In general, the more fiber a food has, the more work your intestines have to do to break it down during digestion. When you are not feeling well and have ulcerative colitis symptoms, you may find that sticking to bland food that doesn't have a lot of fiber and is, therefore, easier to digest helps reduce your discomfort.

Foods that don't leave a lot of undigested material behind in your colon (called low-residue foods) may also be helpful if you are having a flare of ulcerative colitis symptoms. When you have less of this food residue in your intestines, you won't have as many bowel movements.

While the specifics of your ulcerative colitis diet will depend on your individual tastes, preferences, and other dietary needs, choosing foods that can easily move through your intestines without causing too much irritation is a safe bet if you're trying to lessen or prevent symptoms.

RECIPES

Beetroot Tarte Tatin

Ingredients

- 8 small pre-cooked fresh beetroots thickly sliced

- 1 sheet thawed frozen puff pastry

- 8 basil leaves

- 50 grams crumbled feta cheese

- 1 tablespoon brown sugar

- 1 tablespoon balsamic vinegar

- 15 grams butter

Preparation

1. Preheat the oven to 200C fan forced

2. Grease a 24 cm pie tin. Add butter, sugar, vinegar and beetroot to a heavy based fry pan and simmer and stir for approximately 15 mins until the liquid is thick.

3. Beetroots may crumble and the sauce caramelises. Let cool.

4. Place the beetroot pieces into the pie dish and top with pastry. Bake for approximately 25 minutes until the pastry is golden and puffed.

5. When ready remove from oven and let cool for 10 minutes before turning out onto a serving plate. Top the beetroot with basil leaves and crumbled feta.

Turkish Bake

Ingredients

• 250 grams grated zucchini (let the zucchini settle on paper towels to drain excess moisture for 10 minutes, squeeze it a little more to get out the rest of the moisture and then use it)

• ¼ cup chives (finely chopped)

• ½ teaspoon garlic powder

• ¼ cup fresh dill (chopped)

• 1 teaspoon coriander powder

• 1 teaspoon baking powder

• 60 grams white flour

• 120 grams feta cheese crumbled (or vegan feta)

• 3 eggs or vegan easy egg made to specification

• 25 ml extra virgin olive oil

• Salt and pepper to taste

Preparation

1. Preheat the oven to 180C fan forced

2. Grease and line a baking loaf tin with baking paper. In a large bowl mix the chives, zucchini, baking powder, flour, crumbled feta, olive oil, coriander powder, dill herb, and garlic powder and mix thoroughly. Whisk eggs (or egg substitute) and combine evenly with the mixture.

3. Place in the loaf tin and bake for 30 minutes.

4. Remove from oven to check if there is still some moisture in the middle of the loaf by pressing down on the loaf.

5. Return to oven for a further 23-27 minutes or until the mixture is set.

6. Let the loaf stand in the pan for 10 minutes before serving.

7. Serve with lemon wedges, extra dill and mint, Turkish bread and yogurt if desired.

Fresh Fricos

Ingredients

- 750 grams Coliban potatoes (washed and grated)

- 1 tablespoon finely chopped chives

- ½ teaspoon powdered garlic

- 50 mls Extra virgin olive oil

- ½ teaspoon dried rosemary

• 80 grams grated cheese (Montasio if you prefer a more Italian flavour)

• Salt and pepper to taste

Preparation

1. Preheat the oven to 180C fan forced

2. In a large heavy bottomed saucepan add the olive oil and heat to medium, add the onion cook for a minute and add the potato.

3. Continuously toss the potato and onion, and season with salt and pepper.

4. Cook until the potato surfaces are golden and crispy.

5. Grease a 6-hole muffin tray, add the mixture until each hole is full, and press it down into the holes with the back of a spoon.

6. Bake for 20 minutes until the Fricos appear golden

7. Serve with some crispy steamed vegetables with a drizzle of olive oil salt and pepper to taste.

Pho Delicious

Ingredients

• 1000 ml Vietnamese inspired chicken Pho liquid

• 1250 grams skinless chicken thighs (cut into 2.5cm chunks)

- 500 grams (uncooked weight) rice noodles (cooked and ready to add to the soup)

- 5 tablespoons Extra virgin olive oil

- 1 ¼ cup chopped coriander

- 1 ¼ cup mint leaves

- 1 ¼ cup bean sprouts

- 2 ½ lime (quartered)

- 2 ½ peeled julienned carrot

- Salt and pepper to taste

Preparation

1. In a large heavy bottomed saucepan add the olive oil and heat to medium.

2. Add the chunks of chicken and cook until surfaces are brown

3. Let cool for a minute and add stock and bring to the boil then simmer until the chicken is cooked through approximately 15 minutes

4. Warm four bowls

5. Place the cooked noodles in the bowls, add bean sprouts, coriander and mint to each bowl and spoon in the hot soup adding chicken to each dish

6. Decorate with lime quarter.

Zucchini Lasagne

Ingredients

- 800 grams grated zucchini

- 1 teaspoon powdered onion

- 1 teaspoon powdered garlic

- 1 tablespoon chopped chives

- 1 tablespoon dried oregano

- 250 grams low-fat ricotta (or Tofutti*)

- 50 grams fat reduced shredded cheddar (or Sheese*)

- 350 ml passata

- 9 dried lasagne sheets (gluten free if needed*)

- Extra virgin oil

- Salt and pepper to taste

Preparation

1. Preheat the oven to 210C

2. Heat olive oil in a large fry pan and add onion and garlic powder, and zucchini, cook for 3 minutes

3. Turn the heat down and stir in ¾ tub of ricotta and 25 grams of reduced fat cheddar cheese (or vegan versions) add a little salt and pepper to taste – put aside

4. Boil lasagne sheets in water add a pinch of salt for about 5-6 minutes until just soft, but not fully cooked,

drain and add some olive oil to the pasta to stop it sticking and to coat the layers

5. In a baking dish place a layer of lasagne sheet, then ricotta and zucchini mix, sprinkle each layer with oregano and chives, then a layer of tomato passata

6. Repeat layering until all lasagne and mixture is used

7. Add the rest of the ricotta to the top of the lasagne and sprinkle with cheddar cheese (or vegan version)

8. Turn the oven down to 180C

9. Bake the lasagne for 30 minutes until the pasta is soft and the top of the lasagne is golden

10. Serve with salad leaf salad.

Sicilian Pizza

Ingredients

- 4 slices Tortilla bread (or similar)

- 190 grams canned tuna (drained)*

- 2 tablespoons oil (preferably olive oil)

- 90 grams pizza sauce

- 110 grams pitted olives

- 2 finely sliced mushrooms

- 1 cup grated cheese

• Fresh or dried basil leaves

Preparation

1. Preheat the oven to 220C fan forced

2. Drain tuna and break into chunks

3. Top each 'pizza' base with pizza sauce, olives, mushrooms and tuna.

4. Bake for 10 minutes

5. Add cheese to each pizza and bake for a further 5 minutes to melt the cheese.

6. When cooked drizzle olive oil over and sprinkle with dried or fresh basil leaves.

Pasta Bake

Ingredients

• 500 grams peeled pumpkin or sweet potato cut into chunks

• 200 grams tinned asparagus cut into chunks

• 400 grams pasta

• 50 grams white bread broken up into crumbs

• 2 tablespoons oil (preferably olive oil)

• 400 mls vegetable or chicken stock

• 150 grams grated cheese

- 1 teaspoon mixed herbs

Preparation

1. Preheat the oven to 220C (fan forced)

2. Place the pumpkin/sweet potato in a baking dish and drizzle with one tablespoon of olive oil and roast until the vegetables soft and golden

3. At the same time boil the pasta until al dente and drain

4. In a bowl add breadcrumbs, stock, and the rest of the olive oil, mix until breadcrumbs dissolve then add asparagus, pumpkin, mixed herbs, add pasta and mix 100 grams of the cheese through

5. Place in a baking dish and heat through for 30 minutes finish off with the last 50 grams of cheese on top of the dish for 10 minutes until melted

6. Serve with salad or steamed greens.

Nutty Pudding

Ingredients

- 200 grams tinned pear, peach or apple

- 25 grams crushed cashew nuts*

- 1 tablespoon vanilla extract

- Vanilla pod (halved)

- 200 ml whole milk of your choice

- ½ teaspoon allspice mix

- ½ citrus fruit zest

- 75 grams spread of your choice

- 8 slices slightly stale white bread

- 3 free range eggs

- 2 tablespoons sugar or maple syrup or (1 tablespoon of stevia)

- 100 ml cream or coconut cream

Preparation

1. Heat the oven to 180C

2. Gently simmer milk in a small pan add vanilla extract and citrus zest and leave to cool

3. Thinly butter slices of bread on both sides and cut into quarters

4. Mash the fruit in a separate bowl

5. Lay the bread out in the base of the oven dish and add the layer of fruit and crushed nuts

6. Overlap the rest of the bread slices until all slices are used

7. Whip the eggs together with your sugar or sugar substitute add the milk, vanilla and citrus liquid and add cream, whip together until well blended, taste to ensure it is to your desired sweetness

8. Pour over the pudding and leave soak in to 20 minutes

9. Sprinkle the top with all spice

10. Place the oven dish into a roasting tin and fill the roasting tin with water to half way up the side of the pudding dish

11. Cook for 30-40 minutes until pudding is moist but firm

12. Let stand for 5 minutes and serve with vanilla ice cream or yoghurt.

Pesto Salmon

Ingredients

- 4 slices skin on salmon

- 4 ½ slices of fresh lemon

- 1 sprig fresh parsley

- 120 grams pesto

- 200 grams snow peas (trimmed &deveined)

- 2 2 medium carrots (julienned)

- 2 packets white basmati microwavable rice

- Extra virgin olive oil

- Salt and pepper to taste

Preparation

1. Heat the grill to medium.

2. Line a baking tray with foil and lightly baste the foil with olive oil.

3. Put the salmon, skin-side down, on the tray and add some pesto to each piece spreading it evenly across the top.

4. Lightly grill the salmon pieces for about 8 minutes for a pink inside, or longer depending on your preference.

5. Heat the rice as per the packet directions.

6. Lightly steam the carrots and snow peas and add them to the rice and toss through, add another teaspoon of pesto to flavour the grains, salt and pepper to taste.

7. Divide the rice into four bowls and place the salmon on top of each bowl.

8. Squeeze some fresh lemon on top of each piece of salmon and serve with slice of lemon and some parsley leaves.

Winter Apple Poke Bowl

Ingredients

- ½ butternut pumpkin (peeled and chopped)

- 1 red apple (finely sliced)

- 1 sachet precooked basmati rice (microwavable)

- ½ cup chopped chives

- ½ cup parsley and coriander (finely chopped)

- 200 grams haloumi (diced)

- Sprigs of parsley to decorate

- 2 tbsp extra virgin olive oil

- 2 tbsp lemon juice

- 1 tbsp honey

- 1 tsp grated ginger

Preparation

1. Heat an oven to 200C and place butternut pumpkin on baking paper and bake until golden approximately 30-40 minutes

2. Heat a non-stick pan to medium and add haloumi and cook until golden

3. When the pumpkin and haloumi are ready

4. Mix heated heated rice and all the other ingredients together in a bowl, mix through so all the ingredients are evenly distributed

5. Place the rice mix in the bowl and top with pumpkin and haloumi

6. Blend the dressing ingredients together and pour dressing over the top of the salad and garnish with parsley sprig.

Apple Crisps

Ingredients

- 4 red skinned apples (peeled and cored)
- Coconut oil spray
- Cinnamon (optional)

Preparation

1. Preheat the oven to 140C fan forced

2. Slice the apples very thinly through the core to get really thin slices

3. Line a baking tin with baking paper and spray with coconut oil

4. Place the apple slices on the tray do not overlap, spray with coconut oil, if they overlap place extra in separate tray

5. Bake for 40 minutes until the slices are crispy

6. (If you need two trays, at 20minutes into baking swap bottom tray to top tray to ensure equal cooking)

7. Sprinkle with cinnamon

Serving suggestions

1. Float on top of a hot herbal tea

2. Crush and top salads

3. Place on top of chicken or pork dishes

4. Top a breakfast cereal with the crisps for an extra crunch

Miso Apple Soup

Ingredients

- 2000 ml water

- 2 ½ green apple (peeled, cored and grated)

- 500 grams pre cooked rice noodles

- 10 sachet single serve miso paste

- 1 ¼ cup chopped green chives

- 10 finely sliced mushrooms

- 500 grams silken tofu crumbed

- 5 slice crispy roasted seaweed

Preparation

1. Rinse the rice noodles thoroughly in hot water and strain

2. Gently heat water to about 80 degrees

3. Add all ingredients except miso paste and stir for a minute or two until ingredients are warmed through

4. Add the two sachets of miso paste and blend through

5. Top with crushed seaweed flakes.

Fritter Fix

Ingredients

- 350 grams canned tuna or salmon (drained)
- 2 tablespoons oil (preferably olive oil)
- 50 grams tomato paste
- 400 grams cooked white rice (basmati if possible)
- ½ teaspoon paprika
- ½ cup minute oats (optional)
- ¼ cup wholemeal flour
- 1 egg

Preparation

1. Heat the oven to 100C

2. Place rice in a large bowl add minute oats, fish, and paprika and mix thoroughly.

3. Make a well and add the beaten egg and tomato paste and blend until a soft mixture add white flour

4. Form eight fritters

5. Gently heat oil in a pan and add four fritters and cook until golden brown on both sides

6. Place in the oven to keep warm

7. Repeat and cook the last four

8. Serve with a crispy salad and a tablespoon of tomato sauce where possible.

Egg Nests

Ingredients

• 6 free range eggs

• 6 slices white bread

• ¼ cup chopped parsley or (1 tablespoon of dried parsley)

• Extra virgin olive oil

• Ground sea salt and pepper

Preparation

1. Preheat oven to 200C

2. Grease a muffin tray

3. Cut crusts off the bread and press one slice into each muffin mold

4. Place tray into the oven for 5 minutes until bread starts to crisp

5. Beat eggs add chopped/dried parsley

6. Pour eggs evenly into each of the molds and bake until the egg content is firm to the touch (5-10 minutes)

7. Add freshly ground sea salt and pepper to serve.

Sun-Dried Tomato Bacon Mini Frittatas

{Paleo}

Ingredients

* 4 slices sugar free bacon

* 1 cup roughly chopped sundried tomatoes

* 1 and ½ cups roughly chopped broccolini – baby broccoli – florets

* 2 tbsp water

* 8 eggs

* ¼ cup full fat organic canned coconut milk – heavy cream would work too if you tolerate dairy

* ¼ tsp salt

* Generous pinch of black pepper

* 1 tbsp fresh chives finely chopped

Preparation

1. Preheat oven to 375 degrees

2. Preheat a heavy or cast iron skillet to med-hi heat. Chop the bacon crosswise into bite sized pieces and add to the hot pan, stirring as you cook.

3. When the bacon is ¾ of the way done, add the chopped sundried tomatoes to the pan plus the water and stir to coat. Add the chopped broccolini and stir again to coat. Lower the heat to medium and continue to cook for 1 minute before removing from heat.

4. In a large bowl, combine the eggs, coconut milk, salt, black pepper, and chives. Add the bacon mixture to the egg mixture and stir to combine.

5. Grease a muffin pan with coconut oil or extra bacon fat and pour the mixture into each cup ¾ of the way full, so you have 10-12 total filled.

6. Bake in the preheated oven for 15 minutes or until the eggs are just set. Remove and let cool.

7. Either serve warm or store in the fridge, covered, for up to 4 days. Great as a make-ahead dish for brunch, breakfast or as a quick and easy afternoon snack!

8. Enjoy!

Lemon Almond Snack Cake

Ingredients

- 2 cups blanched almond flour

- 1/3 cup tapioca starch

- ½ tsp baking soda

- 1/8 tsp salt

- 3 eggs

- ¾ cup organic coconut sugar

- 3 tbsp coconut oil melted and cooled slightly

- 2 tbsp fresh squeezed lemon juice

- 1 tsp ground ginger

- ½ tsp ground allspice

- 1 and ½ tsp ground cinnamon

Preparation

1. Preheat your oven to 350 degrees and grease an 8 x 8 inch baking dish lightly with coconut oil

2. In a medium bowl, combine the almond flour, tapioca, baking soda, and salt and set aside.

3. In a larger bowl, combine the eggs, coconut sugar, coconut oil, lemon juice, ginger, allspice and cinnamon and beat well

4. Slowly stir the dry ingredients into the wet to fully combine.

5. Transfer the mixture to the prepare baking dish, and bake in the preheated oven for 20-25 minutes or until the top is lightly browned and a toothpick inserted in the center comes out clean.

6. Let cool, then cut into squares and enjoy!

Buttery Dill Mustard Baked Salmon

Ingredients

- 1 6 oz wild caught salmon fillet or 2 if you plan to double!

- 1 tbsp organic ghee clarified butter at room temp (you can use butter if you are fine with dairy)

- 1 tsp brown or dijon mustard

- ½ tsp fresh squeezed lemon juice

- 1 tsp dried dill

- ¼ tsp coarse sea salt

- Pinch of black pepper

Preparation

1. Preheat your oven to 400 degrees

2. Lightly pat the salmon fillet dry on both sides with paper towel to remove excess moisture

3. In a small bowl, combine the ghee or butter, mustard, lemon juice, and dill until smooth

4. Place the salmon in a greased cast iron pan skin side down (or on an aluminum foil covered baking sheet for less cleanup) and sprinkle the top with the sea salt and pepper. Then spread the dill mixture evenly over the top to completely coat.

5. Bake in the preheated oven for 8-10 minutes or until the salmon is cooked through (it will easily flake with a fork when fully cooked)

6. Serve with whatever you want (it's your salmon after all) and enjoy!

Easy Paleo Meatloaf

Ingredients

- 1 lb grassfed ground beef

- 1 lb ground pork

- 1 whole egg

- ¾ tsp salt

- 2 tsp Poultry Seasoning – I used McCormick which includes thyme sage, marjoram, rosemary, black pepper and nutmeg

- ½ tsp dried oregano or 2 tbsp fresh chopped

- ¼ tsp dried basil or 1 tbsp fresh chopped

- 1 tsp dried chives

- ¼ cup maple chipotle ketchup

Preparation

1. Preheat your oven to 400 degrees. In a large bowl, mix the ground meat with the rest of the ingredients until fully combined.

2. Put the entire mixture in a 9 x 5 loaf pan and press down so its evenly distributed, pressing down a bit more in the center for more even baking.

3. Bake in the preheated oven for about 45 minutes or until just no longer pink in the center. Do not overcook! You can test by making a small cut in the very center.

4. Let sit for 5 minutes before slicing and serving over cooked greens or with a side of potatoes. Or both!

Bacon Scallion Chicken Salad

Ingredients

- 1 lb boneless skinless chicken breasts

- 8 slices nitrate free bacon sugar free for Whole30

- ½ cup homemade mayo or Paleo friendly mayo* from Primal Kitchen made with avocado oil

- 2 scallions green onions, thinly sliced

- Salt and pepper to taste

Preparation

1. Take your bacon and chop into bite size pieces. Brown the bacon in a large saute pan over med-hi heat until crisp.

2. Remove bacon from pan and set aside to drain on paper towels, leaving the rendered fat in the pan.

3. Pound the chicken breasts to ½ inch thickness or cut them in half so each piece is ½ inch thick.

4. Turn the heat down to med. Sprinkle the chicken breasts with garlic (if using), salt and pepper and put in the pan with bacon fat. Cook about 2-3 minutes on each side or until the inside is no longer pink.

5. Put the chicken in a large bowl, cover and refrigerate until cool. If you haven't made your mayo yet, now is the time!

6. When the chicken has cooled down, chop roughly into bite size pieces, and in a large bowl, toss together with the bacon, scallions, and mayo. Mix to fully combine.

7. Taste and add salt/pepper if needed. Serve right away or snap a pic for Instagram before you shove the entire bowl in your face. Oh yes, you will!

Peanut Butter Ice Cream

Ingredients

- 4 egg whites

- ⅓ cup white sugar

- 1 cup cream or coconut cream

- 2 tbsp peanut butter

- 2 tbsp icing sugar

- 2 tbsp milk (lactose-free or coconut milk)

Preparation

1. Place the egg whites and the white sugar into the top of a double boiler and heat gently until the sugar has dissolved.

2. Pour into a heatproof bowl and beat to form stiff peaks.

3. Beat the cream in a separate bowl until stiff but not turned.

4. Mix the last 3 ingredients together until a smooth paste is formed.

5. Fold the cream and peanut butter mixture into the egg whites very gently so as not to lose any of the volume. The peanut butter doesn't have to be completely blended. You could leave streaks through the ice cream.

6. Pour into a shallow wide baking pan so the mixture is about 1"/2.5cm deep.

7. Cover with glad wrap and place in the freezer.

8. Once frozen, scoop into bowls or onto ice cream cones to serve.

Curry Dip

Ingredients

- ¼ cup of Greek yoghurt

- ½ cup mayonnaise

- 2 spring onions – green part only
- 1 tsp garam masala
- 1 tsp cumin powder
- 1 tsp coriander powder
- 1 tbsp oil
- 1 tbsp fresh coriander, chopped finely
- 6 drops of hot sauce
- 1 tsp lemon juice
- Salt & pepper

Preparation

1. Heat the oil in a frying pan and add the spring onions chopped finely and the spices.

2. Cook for 1 minute.

3. Add all the ingredients together.

4. Serve with chips or fresh vegetable sticks.

Banana Pancakes

Ingredients

- 1 banana
- 2 eggs
- 1 tsp vanilla essence

- Butter

- Maple syrup

- Raspberries

Preparation

1. Beat the eggs, bananas and vanilla essence together until well blended.

2. Melt a little butter in a frying pan.

3. Once it is bubbling, pour ½ the egg mixture into the pan.

4. Once it is set on one side, flip it over and cook on the other side.

5. Slip out onto a plate and keep warm.

6. Cook the rest of the pancake mixture in the same way,

7. Serve with a few raspberries and a little drizzle of maple syrup.

Jam Cookies

Ingredients

- 2 tbsp olive oil

- ⅓ cup water

- 1 egg

- 1 tbsp maple syrup

- 1 tsp vanilla

- 1 cup tapioca flour

- 2 tbsp coconut flour

- ½ tsp baking soda

- Pinch of salt

- 4 tbsp sugarless strawberry or raspberry jam

Preparation

1. Preheat oven to 180°C/350°F.

2. In a saucepan, mix ⅓ cup tapioca flour, the water and 1 tbsp olive oil. Mix well.

3. Heat on low, stirring until the mixture comes together as a gel.

4. Let it cool.

5. In a bowl, mix the rest of the tapioca flour, the coconut flour, baking soda and salt.

6. Add the slightly beaten egg, 1 tbsp olive oil, maple syrup and vanilla essence. Mix well. It will be quite dry at this point.

7. Add the tapioca gel and knead well together. Add a little more coconut flour if it's too wet or a little water if it's too dry.

8. Roll out between two layers of baking paper.

9. Use a cookie cutter to shape the cookies the way you want them.

10. Gently place on a sheet of baking paper on an oven tray.

11. Bake 5 minutes, turn over and bake 2 minutes.

12. Remove and cool completely.

13. Spread the jam on half the cookies and cover with the rest.

14. Eat while fresh as they will absorb moisture from the air and soften.

Lamb Kofta & Potato Rosti

Ingredients

- 500g/18oz minced lamb
- Small bunch of parsley, chopped
- 1 red chilli, minced
- 1 tsp turmeric
- 1 tsp coriander
- 2 tsp cumin seeds
- Salt & pepper

For the potato rosti:

- 3 large potatoes
- Salt & pepper

- For the sauce:

- 4 tbsp plain yoghurt

- Small bunch of mint, chopped

- 1 tsp cumin powder

- Squeeze of lemon juice

- Salt & pepper

Preparation

For the lamb kofta:

1. Mix all the ingredients together.

2. Shape into a long sausage and insert a wooden skewer.

3. Place on a heated, oiled grill and cook until cooked, turning a few times.

For the potato rosti:

1. Peel the potatoes.

2. Pass them through the grate function of a food processor.

3. Squeeze all the liquid out of the grated potato with your hands.

4. Season with salt and pepper.

5. Heat a mixture of oil and butter in a frying pan.

6. Place big spoonfuls of the potato in the pan and flatten as well as shape them into round shapes.

7. Cook well until browned, then turn and cook on the other side. Don't have the heat too high or they will brown before they are cooked through.

8. Remove from the pan and place on paper towels to absorb some of the oil.

For the sauce:

1. Combine all of the ingredients and place in a small bowl to serve with the lamb.

Lemon Marshmallow Slice

Ingredients

For the base:

- 1 cup of my gluten-free flour blend

- 2 tsp cane sugar

- Pinch of salt

- 80gms/2.75oz chilled butter

- 1 egg

- 2 tsp cider vinegar

For the lemon layer:

- 400mls/13.5oz cream

- 3 tbsp cane sugar

- ⅓ cup lemon juice

- 2 tbsp gelatin

- 1 tbsp tapioca flour

For the marshmallow:

- 2 tbsp gelatin

- ¼ cup water

- 1.5cups cane sugar

- 1 cup water

- 1 tsp vanilla

Preparation

For the base:

1. Preheat the oven to 180°C/350°F.

2. In a food processor, add the flour, sugar, salt and butter, cut up small.

3. Process until crumbs form.

4. Whisk together the egg and vinegar.

5. Add to the processor and process again until a firm dough forms.

6. Adjust with a little cold water or a little more flour if necessary to get a dough which stays together but doesn't crumble.

7. Butter and line a 17.5 x 27.5cm/7" x 11" slice tin.

8. Press the dough into the prepared tin.

9. Place in the oven for 10 minutes or until golden.

10. Cool completely.

For the lemon layer:

1. Bring the cream and sugar to the boil.

2. Add the lemon juice and stir.

3. Dissolve the gelatine in a little hot water and add. Whisk.

4. Mix the tapioca flour in a little cold water and add.

5. Keep stirring until it thickens then take off the heat and let cool.

6. Pour it over the cooled base.

7. Place in the fridge to set completely.

For the marshmallow:

1. Place everything in a saucepan and bring to the boil, stirring.

2. Let boil, not stirring, for 15 minutes.

3. Cool to lukewarm.

4. With egg beaters or a stand mixer, whisk until thick and white.

5. Pour onto the set lemon layer and place in the fridge to firm up.

6. Once set completely, cut into slices.

Potato Fish Cakes

Ingredients

- 2 large potatoes
- 400gms/14oz fish
- 100gms/4oz spinach
- 2 eggs
- 2 tbsp tapioca flour
- Squeeze of lemon
- Salt & pepper

Preparation

1. Preheat the oven to 350°F/180°C.

2. Boil the potatoes and puree in a food processor.

3. Chop the spinach finely in the food processor.

4. Mince the fish in the food processor.

5. Mix them all in a bowl with the eggs and flour.

6. Season and add the lemon juice.

7. Heat some butter in a frying pan and add big spoonfuls of the mixture.

8. Shape into circles when in the pan.

9. When browned on both sides, place in an oiled ovenproof dish and pop some cheese on top, if you like.

10. Place in the oven for 10 minutes.

11. Serve with your favourite sauce and a few sprouts or greens.

Pita Bread & Mexican Spread

Ingredients

For the pita bread:

- 1 egg

- 2 tbsp olive oil

- 5 tbsp water

- ¼ tsp salt

- 1 cup tapioca flour

- ½ tsp baking soda

- 1 tsp cumin seeds

For the mince:

- 400gms/14oz minced beef

- 2 tbsp oil

- 1 carrot

- 1 stick of celery

- 1 courgette

- 1 tsp cumin

- 1 tsp garam marsala

- 1 tsp coriander powder

- ½ tsp turmeric

- Salt & pepper

- ¾ cup water

- 1 tbsp tapioca flour

- Squeeze of lemon juice

- Chopped mint

For the avocado:

- 1 avocado

- 2 heaped tbsp creme fraiche

- 2 tsp lemon juice

- Salt & pepper

To serve:

- 2 chopped tomatoes

- A small pot of sour cream

Preparation

For the pita bread:

1. Preheat the oven to 375 degrees F or 190 degrees C.

2. In a pot, mix ⅓ cup of flour, water and 1 tbsp olive oil.

3. Heat on low, stirring, until the mixture completely sticks together.

4. Take off the heat and let cool.

5. In a bowl, mix the rest of the flour, baking soda and salt.

6. Add the egg and the rest of the oil.

7. Add the cooled congealed mixture and knead together into a dough.

8. Push it out into a flat, round shape on a baking tray which has been covered with baking paper.

9. Bake until crisp on one side (around 20 minutes)and then turn over and crisp up on that side too (another 5 minutes).

10. Remove from the oven and cut into wedges.

For the mince:

1. Peel the carrot and courgette and chop roughly with the celery.

2. Place in a food processor and chop small.

3. Heat the oil in a frying pan and add all the spices. Heat to release the aromas.

4. Add the minced vegetables and cook for 5 minutes.

5. Add the mince and cook until well browned.

6. Season.

7. Add the water and the tapioca flour dissolved in a little water.

8. Stir to blend and thicken.

9. Squeeze over half a lemon and mix.

10. Remove from the heat and serve with a sprinkle of mint.

For the avocado:

1. Mash all the ingredients together and serve with the mince, pita bread, tomatoes and sour cream.

Coconut Chocolate Whoopie Pies

Ingredients

For the cookies:

• ¼ cup coconut flour

• ½ cup oil

• 2-3 tbsp date puree (depends how sweet you want your cookies)

• 1 ripe banana

• 2 eggs

• 1 tsp cinnamon

• 1 tsp vanilla

• Pinch salt

- ½ tsp baking soda

- 1 cup of coconut

For the filling:

- ½ cup coconut cream

- 150g /5oz sugarless chocolate

Preparation

For the cookies:

1. Heat the oven to 350°F/180°C.

2. Mix the flour, butter and date puree in a food processor.

3. Add the eggs and vanilla and mix.

4. Add all other ingredients except the coconut.

5. Remove the mixture from the food processor to a bowl and add the coconut.

6. Place a sheet of baking paper on an oven tray.

7. Drop big spoonfuls of the dough onto the paper and shape them into circles.

8. Bake about 10 minutes until they are golden but still soft.

9. Remove from the oven and leave to cool on the tray for half an hour so they firm up a little.

For the filling:

1. Heat the coconut cream gently in a saucepan.

2. Break up the chocolate into smallish pieces.

3. Pour the hot cream over the chocolate and let it stand for a while.

4. Stir vigorously to a smooth paste.

5. If there are still pieces of unmelted chocolate, place in the microwave for 20

6. Seconds and stir again.

7. Place in the fridge to firm up – about 15 minutes.

8. Pipe the chocolate ganache onto half the cookies and cover with the remaining cookies.

Potato Rosti Pizza

Ingredients

- 4 potatoes, peeled

- Salt & pepper

- A bag of spinach

- 1 tomato

- Edam cheese or mozzarella

- Coconut oil & butter

Preparation

1. Preheat the oven to 180°C/350°F.

2. Grate the potatoes in a food processor or with a hand grater.

3. Squeeze out all the water and dry with a clean tea towel.

4. Season with salt and pepper and mix well.

5. Melt the butter and coconut oil in a frying pan.

6. Place heaped spoonfuls of the mixture into the hot oil/butter mixture and shape into rough, flat circles.

7. Fry until golden on both sides.

8. Meanwhile wilt the spinach in another frying pan with a little butter.

9. Place the cooked rosti on baking paper on a baking tray.

10. Place a layer of spinach on top of each one.

11. Follow with a slice of tomato and season.

12. Layer a slice of cheese on top and place the tray in the oven for about 5 minutes until the cheese is melted.

Summer Squash Soup

Ingredients:

• 3 tablespoons Garlic-Infused Oil, made with vegetable oil or olive oil, or purchased equivalent

• 1 cup (64 g) finely chopped scallions, green parts only

- 4 cups (600 g) chopped trimmed patty pan squash

- 4 medium Yukon gold potatoes, peeled and chopped

- 3 medium carrots, trimmed, peeled and chopped

- 1 teaspoon cumin powder

- 1 teaspoon coriander

- 1 teaspoon turmeric

- 1 teaspoon paprika, plus extra for garnish

- ¼ teaspoon mustard powder

- ¼ teaspoon cinnamon

- 4 ½ cups (1 L) Vegetable Broth

- ¾ cup (180 ml) canned whole coconut milk, at room temperature

- Kosher salt

- Freshly ground black pepper

- Cilantro leaves

Preparation:

1. Heat a large, heavy-bottomed pot over low-medium heat. Add the oil and the scallion greens and sauté until softened, but not browned. Add the squash, potatoes, carrots and all of the spices. Stir together and cook for a few minutes or until vegetables just begin to soften. Add the stock, cover, bring to a boil, then adjust heat and simmer for about 15 minutes or until all the vegetables are very tender.

2. If you have an immersion blender, you can purée the soup right in the pot. Otherwise, transfer to blender and purée. Return soup to pot, if necessary. Taste and season with salt and pepper. Soup is ready to garnish and serve. Divide the hot soup into serving bowls, swirl in some coconut milk, garnish with cilantro leaves and a sprinkle of paprika. You can also refrigerate the puréed soup in an airtight container (before garnishing) for up to 4 days.

One-Bowl Streusel Coffeecake

Ingredients:

Streusel:

• 4 tablespoons (½ stick; 57 g) unsalted butter, cut into pieces

• ⅓ cup (65 g) sugar

• Teaspoons cinnamon

• ¼ teaspoon salt

• ¾ cup (109 g) gluten-free all-purpose flour, such as Bob's Red Mill 1 to 1 Gluten Free Baking Flour

Cake:

• ½ cup (1 stick; 113 g) unsalted butter, at room temperature, cut into pieces

• ⅔ cup (131 g) sugar

• teaspoons vanilla extract

• 2 large eggs, at room temperature

• 1 ¾ cups (254 g) gluten-free all-purpose flour, such as Bob's Red Mill 1 to 1 Gluten-Free Baking Flour

• teaspoons baking powder; use gluten-free if following a gluten-free diet

• ½ teaspoon salt

• 1 cup (240 ml) lactose-free whole milk, at room temperature

Preparation:

1. Position rack in center of oven. Preheat oven to 350°F (180°C). Coat the insides of an 8-inch (20 cm) square cake pan with nonstick spray; set aside.

2. For the Streusel: Melt the butter in a large microwave safe bowl. Whisk in the sugar, cinnamon and salt then stir in the flour until clumps form; set aside on a piece of parchment. No need to wash out bowl (the streusel should come out of the bowl very cleanly).

3. For the Cake: Using same bowl, melt the butter, then whisk in sugar and vanilla. Now whisk in eggs one at a time. Add flour, bajing powder and salt and begin to stir/fold everything together with a sturdy wooden spoon or silicone spatula until partway combined. Add milk, switch to a whisk and continue to beat until you get a fluid batter.

4. Scrape about half of the batter into the prepared pan (you can do this by eye). Scatter about ½ cup of the streusel evenly over the batter, squeezing it into clumps

as you go (this is about a handful). Top with remaining batter, gently spreading into an even layer. Top evenly with remaining streusel.

5. Bake for about 25 to 35 minutes or until a toothpick shows a few moist crumbs clinging. The cake will have begun to come away from the sides of the pan and the streusel will be golden. Cool on rack for at least 10 minutes. Cut into a 4 by 4 grid to make 16 servings and serve warm, or at room temperature. Cake may be stored at room temperature overnight, well wrapped with plastic wrap.

Instant Pot Caribbean-Style Pork

Ingredients:

- ½ cups (375 g) finely chopped fresh pineapple, with all juices

- 1 cup (64 g) finely chopped scallions, green parts only

- ½- ounce (127 g) can mild green chiles, such as Hatch

- 1 ½ tablespoons unsulphured molasses

- 1 tablespoon low FODMAP hot sauce, such as Tabasco

- 1 teaspoon FreeFod Garlic Replacer

- 1 teaspoon FreeFod Onion Replacer

- 1 teaspoon ground ginger

- 1 teaspoon kosher salt

- 1 teaspoon dried thyme

- ½ teaspoon ground allspice

- ½ teaspoon freshly ground black pepper

- ½ teaspoon freshly grated nutmeg

- ½ teaspoon turmeric

- 1 Pound to 3 ½-pound (1.4 kg to 1.6 kg) bone-in or boneless pork butt or shoulder, at room temperature

Preparation:

1. Stir together the pineapple, scallion greens, chiles, molasses, hot sauce, the FreeFod Garlic Replacer and the FreeFod Onion Replacer, ginger, salt, thyme, allspice, black pepper and nutmeg in your Instant Pot.

2. Add the pork and turn to coat. Lock the lid in place. Set the Instant Pot to Pressure Cook on Maximum for 1 hour 10 minutes with the Keep Warm setting off. Press Start. Allow the pot to cook and then return to normal pressure on its own, which will take about 20 to 30 minutes after the timed cooking period. Unlock the lid. Remove the pork to a large bowl, where you can shred it with two forks.

3. Skim excess fat off of the surface of the sauce and discard. Set machine to Sauté on Medium/Normal/Custom 300°F (150°C) for 20 minutes and press Start. It will come to a simmer. Keep an eye on it, stir occasionally, and reduce it until it thickens. Re-combine the sauce with the meat, tossing together thoroughly. Taste and adjust seasoning at this time. Your

pork is ready to serve, perhaps with a side of rice or fried plantains.

Instant Pot Chicken Noodle Soup

Ingredients:

• 2tablespoons Garlic-Infused Oil, Onion-Infused Oil or olive oil

• 1 cup (64 g) finely chopped scallions, green parts only

• ½ cup (36 g) very finely chopped leeks, green parts only

• 2 medium carrots, trimmed, peeled and chopped into large bite-size pieces

• 2 medium parsnips, trimmed, peeled and chopped into large bite-size pieces

• 1 medium stalk celery, trimmed and chopped into large bite-size pieces

• 6 cups (1.4 L) Chicken Stock, homemade or purchased

• 1Pound (455 g) boneless, skinless chicken breast, cut into 4 pieces

• 2 medium-sized skinless bone-in chicken thighs

• 2 tablespoons chopped fresh flat-leaf parsley

• ½ teaspoons dried thyme

• 1 bay leaf

- Kosher salt

- Freshly ground black pepper

- 5- ounces (140 g) gluten-free egg noodles, such as Jovial Tagliatelle

- Fresh dill; optional

Preparation:

1. Press Instant Pot button for "Sauté" and set the temperature to High for 10 minutes. Add oil, scallions, leeks, carrots, parsnips and celery and sauté for 10 minutes or until beginning to soften. Stop the machine.

2. Set your Instant Pot to Pressure Cook/Soup/High for 10 minutes. Add stock, chicken, parsley, thyme and bay leaf, lock lid and press Start. Allow to come to normal pressure naturally. Remove the chicken, discard the bones and shred or chop the flesh into bite sized pieces; set aside.

3. Turn the Sauté function on High and bring soup to a simmer. Add pasta and cook till tender, stirring occasionally. Add the boneless chicken back to pot. Remove bay leaf, taste and season with salt and pepper.

One Pan Roast

Ingredients

- 1 individual red potato peeled and chopped

- 1 kg sweet potato peeled and chopped

- 1 large red capsicum halved, skin removed and deseeded and chopped

- 4 accorn squash halved

- 300 grams green beans

- 6 chicken sausages chopped into 2cm slices(or vegan/gluten free)

- 1 large zucchini chopped

- 1 teaspoon powdered garlic

- 1 tablespoon dried parsley

- 1 tablespoon died oregano

- 1 teaspoon smokey paprika

- Salt and pepper to taste

- Extra virgin oil for basting

- 1 tablespoon chopped leaf fresh parsley (no stalks)

Preparation

1. Preheat the oven to 180C

2. Line the pan with baking paper

3. Add all the vegetables and herbs into a large bowl and add 4 tablespoons of olive oil and mix the vegetables and sausage thoroughly through to coat them with herbs and oil

4. Place on a baking tray and bake for 15 minutes and toss the vegetables around and bake for a further 15-20 minutes until vegetables are soft and browned

5. Serve immediately or refrigerate and serve cold the next day

6. Serve with quinoa or brown rice.

Pumpduken

Ingredients

- 1cup milk

- 2kg peeled butternut pumpkin

- 1/3 cup smooth peanut butter

- ½ cup cooked basmati rice

- 2teablespoons chopped chives

- 1teaspoon dried garlic

- 100 grams crumbled feta

- 1 beaten egg

- 2teaspon chopped rosemary leaves

- 1large red capsicum halved and deseeded

- 1 long zucchini halved and deseeded (to make a well in each side)

- ½ cup carrot finely chopped

- String to tie the pumpduken

- Tomato passata with a dash of Worcestershire sauce to serve

- Extra virgin olive oil for basting

Preparation

1. Preheat the oven to 180C

2. Cut the peeled pumpkin in half and bake for 20 minutes until tender, take out of the oven

3. Scrape the middle out of each pumpkin half to make a well leaving a 2 cms thick outer wall of the pumpkin for the inner ingredients, set aside

4. In a heavy bottomed pan heat some olive oil, soften add dried garlic and chives stir through then add rosemary leaves

5. Mix rice, onion, garlic, fetta, and egg in a large bowl

6. Press the mixture down inside the pumpkin, leave a little of the mixture for packing around the inner vegetables

7. Press the capsicum halves, one in each side of the pumpkin and press down

8. Mix chopped carrot and smooth peanut butter together in a bowl

9. Place a zucchini half inside the capsicum and fill with chopped carrot and peanut butter mixture

10. Fill the remaining space between the capsicum and zucchini with the last of the rice mixture

11. Press everything down and gently place two halves of the pumpkin together and tie with string to keep together

12. Place on a baking tray and bake for 50-60 minutes until pumpkin is soft to touch

13. Gently remove the string and cut into slices and serve on with tomato salsa.

Twisted Tomato Soup

Ingredients

- 2kilo large tomatoes de seeded and *peeled

- 20grams tomato paste

- 750ml salt reduced Massel chicken style stock

- 100grams plain greek yoghurt

- 1tablespoon onion powder

- 1tablespoon granulated garlic

- 30 ml extra virgin olive oil

- 2tablespoons balsamic vinegar

- 1teaspoon fresh thyme leaves

- Cracked salt and pepper to taste

• Extra olive oil to drizzle on top of soup

Preparation

1. Preheat oven to 200C

2. Halve tomatoes

3. Oil a baking tray with half of the olive oil

4. Place tomatoes on the tray and sprinkle with onion powder and garlic granules

5. Mix remaining olive oil and balsamic vinegar and drizzle over the tomatoes

6. Sprinkle with thyme leaves, season with salt and pepper

7. Bake for 30 minutes until the tomatoes are partially caramelised (browned)

8. Remove from tray and place into a large pot, adding stock and then simmer for 10 minutes, take off heat

9. Carefully blend soup until completely smooth

10. Just before serving mix yoghurt through

11. Place in individual bowls

12. Drizzle a little extra olive oil on top before serving

13. Serve with crusty rustic wholemeal wholegrain bread.

Caprese Bocconcini Skewers

Ingredients

- 220grams Bambini (or cherry) bocconcini

- Basil leaves

- 16 x 2cm cubes watermelon (no seeds)

- Balsamic glaze

- Wooden skewers

Preparation

1. Skewer melon ball first then a folded basil leaf then a bocconcini ball, followed by another folded basil leaf and a final melon ball

2. Lie skewers flat on a long dish and repeat until all ingredients are used

3. Drizzle a zig zag of balsamic glaze down the centre of the skewers and serve.

Pulao Rice Prawns

Ingredients

- 50fresh deveined shelled prawns

- 8tablespoon extra virgin olive oil

- 1250ml water

- 500ml coconut milk

- 8cardamoms

- 2bay leaves

- ½pinch red chilli powder

- ¼teaspoon turmeric powder

- 2/3cup chopped coriander

- Black pepper

- Himalayan salt

- Garam masala powder

- ½ pinch asafoetida powder

Preparation

1. Heat olive oil in a thick bottomed pan and add the spices clove, bay leaves, cardamoms and a generous few grinds of black pepper cook until fragrant 1-2 minutes

2. Place the cloves, bay leaves, cardamoms in a tea leaf ball (yes the ones that you put tea leaves in for a cup of tea – this is to stop the whole herbs being problematic in the bowel but to let them release their flavour)

3. Add the prawns, salt, chilli powder, garam masala, turmeric and asafoetida and mix well

4. Drain and add rice to the pan and mix well with 500ml of water and 200ml of coconut milk

5. Turn the heat down and simmer until the rice is completely cooked

6. Toss through fresh coriander just before serving

7. Serve with blanched deveined snow peas.

Creamy Cherry Smoothie

Ingredients

- ¼ripe avocado

- 100ml dark cherry juice

- 1teaspoon hulled tahini

- 1teaspoon lecithin granules

- 150ml unsweetened oat milk

- 1tablespoon coconut crème

- 1Maraschino cherry (optional to serve)

Preparation

1. Add all ingredients and blend until smooth

2. Serve with a split maraschino cherry on the side of the glass.

Lemon Baked Eggs

Ingredients

- 2grams large free range eggs

- 2slices low fat cheddar cheese

- 1teaspoon salt preserved lemon julienned

- 2tablespoon chopped parsley

- Extra virgin olive oil spray

- 1crusty white roll to serve

Preparation

1. Heat the oven at 180 C

2. Spray a small single serve soufflé dish with olive oil

3. Cut the cheddar cheese into three lengthways strips and line the outer inside edges of the dish with the cheese you can double line if any left over

4. Crack the eggs into the centre

5. Gently place the thin strips of julienned lemon on top of the eggs with a sprinkle of parsley

6. Place the dish in the oven and cook for eight to ten minutes and check them

7. If you want them firmer cook for another 2-3 minutes

8. Sprinkle the top of the eggs with more parsley

9. Serve with hot crusty white bread rolls.

Orange French Toast

Ingredients

French Toast

- 1 large egg
- 2 tsp. Grand Marnier orange liqueur
- ½ tsp. Sugar
- 1 Tbsp. 2% milk
- ¼ tsp. Pure vanilla extract
- ¼ cup orange juice
- ¼ tsp. Orange zest
- 4 slices sourdough bread
- 2 tsp. (per serving) unsalted butter

Orange Honey

- 2 Tbsp. Honey
- ½ tsp. Grand Marnier orange liqueur

Preparation

1. Place the egg, Grand Marnier, sugar, milk, vanilla extract, orange juice, and orange peel in a medium mixing bowl.

2. Whisk until well blended.

3. Heat a non-stick griddle over medium-high heat.

4. When the griddle is hot enough that a few drops of water will dance on the surface, reduce the heat to medium and place 4 slices of bread into the batter.

5. Gently dunk and turn the bread until it is well coated and slightly soaked.

6. Place the 4 slices of soaked bread on the griddle and cook for about 3 – 4 minutes. Turn and cook on the other side.

7. Cook, turning occasionally, until both sides are golden brown.

8. Depending on your stove or griddle you may need to reduce the heat slightly.

9. Remove and top with the butter and orange honey.

Orange Blueberry Scones

Ingredients

- 2 cups all purpose flour

- ¼ cup light brown sugar

- 2 tsp baking powder

- ½ tsp salt

- 2 Tbsp unsalted butter (softened)

- 1 tsp fresh grated orange peel

- ¼ cup orange juice

- ¾ cup non-fat buttermilk

- ¼ cup blueberries

- 2 Tbsp non-fat buttermilk

- 1 Tbsp light brown sugar

Preparation

1. Preheat oven to 425F.

2. Sift the flour, brown sugar, baking powder and salt into a large mixing bowl.

3. Cut in the softened butter with the tines of a fork or a pastry knife. It is well blended when the mixture is the consistency of coarse corn meal.

4. Add the orange juice and orange peel slowly while kneading the batter (I use a rubber spatula). Continue kneading while adding the buttermilk. The mixture will become a sticky dough.

5. Gently fold in the blueberries taking care not to let any burst.

6. Divide the dough into eight small triangles onto a non-stick cookie sheet.

7. Mix together the 2 Tbsp. Buttermilk and 1 Tbsp. Brown sugar and gently wash the tops of the scones. Place in the oven and bake for about 15 – 18 minutes until the tops of the scones are golden.

Pan Grilled Tenderloin with Beurre Bercy

Ingredients

- 1 small shallot (minced)

- 2 cups no salt added beef or vegetable stock

- ¼ tsp salt

- ½ cup white wine

- 1 tap fresh ground black pepper

- 1 Tbsp unsalted butter

- 2 4-ounce beef tenderloin filets

- Spray olive oil

Preparation

1. Place the minced shallot, stock, salt, white wine and fresh ground black pepper in a small sauce pan.

2. Cook for about 30 minutes over medium-high heat until the liquid is completely reduced.

3. Swirl occasionally.

4. The finished reduction should be a thick sauce with barely any liquid left.

5. Remove from the heat and allow to cool for about ten minutes.

6. Add the butter whisking as it melts to incorporate this into the shallot/pepper reduction. Set aside.

7. Preheat the oven to 450°F. Place a non-stick grill pan in the oven and allow it to heat for about ten minutes.

8. Lightly spritz the pan with olive oil and add the filet. Cook on the first side for 5 – 7 minutes.

9. Turn and cook for about another 4 – 5 minutes for rare and 6 – 7 minutes for medium rare.

10. Remove and place on plate.

11. Top with one tablespoon sauce and serve.

Pasta with Sauce Bolognese

Ingredients

• 1 tsp. Olive oil

• 1 medium onion (diced)

• 2 medium carrots (diced)

• 2 cloves garlic (minced)

• 8 ounces lean ground beef (90/10)

• 2 ½ cups water

• ¼ tsp. Salt

• To taste fresh ground black pepper

• 1/8 tsp. Dried tarragon

• 1/8 tsp. Dried thyme

- 2 bay leaves

- ½ tsp. Dried oregano

- ½ tsp. Dried sage

- 3 Tbsp. No salt added tomato paste

- 1 Tbsp. Worcestershire sauce

- 4 quarts water

- 4 ounces whole wheat or gluten free spaghetti, capellini, or fettuccine

Preparation

1. Place the olive oil in a medium skillet over medium-high heat.

2. Add the onion, carrots, and garlic.

3. Reduce the heat to medium and cook, stirring frequently, until the onion has softened slightly.

4. Add the ground beef.

5. Cook until the beef is browned. Stir frequently.

6. Add the water, salt, pepper, tarragon, thyme, bay leaves, oregano, and sage.

7. Reduce the heat to medium-low and cook, stirring occasionally, for two hours. Each time you stir, gently mash the carrots with the back of a spoon to crush them. If the liquid reduces below about ½ cup, add water ¼ cup at a time.

8. After the sauce has simmered for two hours, add the tomato paste and Worcestershire sauce.

9. Stir and simmer 15 minutes while you make the pasta (below).

10. When the sauce is nearly done, place the water in a large sauce pan over high heat. When it boils add the pasta and cook until it is just tender. Drain the pasta and add it to the sauce. Cook over low heat, tossing frequently, for about 2 minutes. Serve.

Roast Tenderloin with Merlot Blackberry

Sauce

Ingredients

- 2 cups merlot

- 1 pint fresh blackberries

- 1 cup low sodium chicken or vegetable broth

- ¼ tsp salt

- 1/8 tsp fresh ground black pepper

- ¼ tsp dried thyme

- 2 Tbsp maple syrup

- 2 Tbsp unsalted butter

- 4 ounce tenderloin filets

- Spray olive oil

- 1/8 tsp salt

- Fresh ground black pepper

- Tenderloin with wine sauce

Preparation

1. Place the merlot, blackberries, chicken stock, salt, pepper, thyme and maple syrup in a medium stainless or non-reactive sauce pan. Place the pan over high heat and bring to a boil. Reduce the heat to low and simmer for 30 minutes.

2. Use a potato masher or a slotted spoon to gently mash all of the blackberries. Cook on simmer for another 15 minutes.

3. Strain the sauce through a fine mesh strainer. Press down with a rubber spatula to remove all the liquid. Discard the pulp and seeds.

4. Rinse the sauce pan and return the strained sauce. Simmer for another 15 minutes until reduced by half. There should be about ½ to 2/3 cup sauce. Add 2 tablespoons butter and whisk until dissolved. Set aside.

5. Heat a large non-stick skillet over medium-high heat. When hot spray lightly with the oil and add the filets. Sprinkle the tops lightly with the salt and pepper. Cook for about 5- 7 minute and turn. Cook for another 5 minutes for rare to medium rare.

6. Serve topped with 2 tablespoons warm sauce.

Asparagus Frittata

Ingredients

- 1 tsp unsalted butter
- ¼ cup onion (diced)
- 2 asparagus spears
- 2 large eggs
- 2 large egg whites
- 2 Tbsp water
- 4 Tbsp Parmigiano-Reggiano (grated)
- Fresh ground black pepper (to taste)

Preparation

1. Preheat the oven to 400F.

2. Heat ½ teaspoon butter in a small non-stick sauteed pan over low-medium heat and add the chopped onion. Cook until translucent and set aside.

3. Slice the base of asparagus crosswise into small rounds. Leave about 2 inches of the tops intact. Set the tops aside to decorate the top of the frittata.

4. Whisk the eggs, egg whites and water in a bowl until frothy.

5. Heat the remaining butter in a small non-stick skillet over medium- high heat and when hot add the egg mixture. Reduce the heat to medium and simmer for

about 2 minutes. At the end of one minute add the onion and chopped asparagus.

6. Arrange the asparagus tops in a star pattern on top of the cooking egg mixture. Scatter the parmesan cheese over the top and then fresh ground black pepper to taste.

7. Place in the oven. Reduce the heat to 350F degrees and bake for 10 – 15 minutes until it puffs and is firm to the touch.

Chipotle spiced shrimp

Ingredients

- 1 pound uncooked shrimp, peeled and deveined

- 2 tablespoons tomato paste

- 1 ½ teaspoons water

- ½ teaspoon extra-virgin olive oil

- ½ teaspoon minced garlic

- ½ teaspoon chipotle chili powder

- ½ teaspoon chopped fresh oregano

Preparation

1. Rinse shrimp in cold water. Pat dry with a paper towel and set aside on a plate.

2. To make the marinade, in a small bowl, whisk together the tomato paste, water and oil. Add garlic, chili powder and oregano. Mix well.

3. Using a brush, spread the marinade (it will be thick) on both sides of the shrimp. Place in the refrigerator.

4. Prepare a hot fire in a charcoal grill or heat a gas grill or broiler. Away from the heat source, lightly coat the grill rack or broiler pan with cooking spray. Position the cooking rack 4 to 6 inches from the heat source.

5. Put the shrimp in a grill basket or on skewers and place on the grill. Turn the shrimp after 3 to 4 minutes. The cooking time varies depending on the heat of the fire, so watch carefully.

6. Transfer to a plate and serve immediately.

Ginger-marinated grilled portobello mushrooms

Ingredients

- ¼ cup balsamic vinegar

- ½ cup pineapple juice

- 2 tablespoons chopped fresh ginger, peeled

- 4 large portobello mushrooms (about 4 ounces each), cleaned and stems removed

• 1 tablespoon chopped fresh basil

Preparation

1. In a small bowl, whisk together the balsamic vinegar, pineapple juice and ginger.

2. Place the mushrooms in a glass dish, stemless side up. Drizzle the marinade over the mushrooms. Cover and marinate in the refrigerator for about 1 hour, turning mushrooms once.

3. Prepare a hot fire in a charcoal grill or heat a gas grill or broiler. Away from the heat source, lightly coat the grill rack or broiler pan with cooking spray. Position the cooking rack 4 to 6 inches from the heat source.

4. Grill or broil the mushrooms on medium heat, turning often, until tender, about 5 minutes on each side. Baste with marinade to keep from drying out.

5. Using tongs, transfer the mushrooms to a serving platter. Garnish with basil and serve immediately.

Marinated Portobello Mushrooms With

Provolone

Ingredients

• 2 portobello mushrooms, stemmed and wiped clean

• ½ cup balsamic vinegar

- 1 tablespoon brown sugar

- ¼ teaspoon dried rosemary

- 1 teaspoon minced garlic

- ¼ cup grated (1 ounce) provolone cheese

Preparation

1. Heat the broiler (grill). Position the rack 4 inches from the heat source. Lightly coat a glass baking dish with cooking spray. Place the mushrooms in the dish, stemless-side (gill-side) up.

2. In a small bowl, whisk together the vinegar, brown sugar, rosemary and garlic. Pour the mixture over the mushrooms. Set aside for 5 to 10 minutes to marinate.

3. Broil (grill) the mushrooms, turning once, until they're tender, about 4 minutes on each side. Sprinkle grated cheese over each mushroom and continue to broil (grill) until the cheese melts. Transfer to individual plates.

Roasted Potatoes With Garlic And Herbs

Ingredients

- ¾ pound small (2-inch) white or red potatoes

- 4 garlic cloves

- 2 teaspoons olive oil

- 2 teaspoons chopped fresh rosemary

- 1/8 teaspoon salt

- ¼ teaspoon ground black pepper

- 2 teaspoons butter

- 2 tablespoons chopped fresh parsley

Preparation

1. Heat oven to 400 F. Lightly coat a large baking dish with cooking spray.

2. In a large mixing bowl, add the whole potatoes, garlic cloves, olive oil, rosemary, salt and pepper. Use your hands to mix until the potatoes are coated with the oil and spices.

3. Arrange the potatoes in a single layer in the prepared baking dish. Cover with a lid or aluminum foil and bake for 25 minutes.

4. Remove the lid or foil. Turn potatoes and bake uncovered until the potatoes are soft and slightly browned, about 25 minutes.

5. Transfer to a serving bowl and mix with butter. Sprinkle with parsley and serve.

Strawberry Banana Milkshake

Ingredients

- 6 frozen strawberries, chopped

- 1 medium banana

- ½ cup soy milk

- 1 cup fat-free vanilla frozen yogurt

- 2 fresh strawberries, sliced

Preparation

1. In a blender, combine the frozen strawberries, banana, soy milk and frozen yogurt. Blend until smooth.

2. Pour into tall, frosty glasses and garnish each with fresh strawberry slices. Serve immediately.

Pork And Mushroom Casserole With Gremolata

Ingredients

- 2 tablespoons plain flour

- 1kg boneless pork shoulder, trimmed, cut into 3cm pieces

- 2 tablespoons extra virgin olive oil

- 1 brown onion, thinly sliced

- 2 celery stalks, chopped

- 2 garlic cloves, thinly sliced

- 500g Swiss brown mushrooms, thickly sliced

- 1 tablespoon roughly chopped fresh rosemary

- 1 tablespoon roughly chopped fresh sage leaves

- 1 tablespoon roughly chopped fresh thyme leaves

- 1 ½ cups Massel salt reduced chicken style liquid stock

- ¾ cup pearl barley

- 2 tablespoons chopped fresh flat-leaf parsley leaves

- 2 teaspoons lemon zest

- 2 bunches steamed broccolini, to serve

Preparation

1. Preheat oven to 180C/160C fan-forced.

2. Place flour in a snap-lock bag. Season with pepper. Add pork. Seal bag. Shake to coat. Heat ½ the oil in a large, flameproof casserole dish over high heat. Cook pork, in batches, for 5 minutes or until browned, adding more oil if needed. Transfer to a plate.

3. Heat remaining oil in dish over medium-high heat. Add onion, celery, garlic, mushroom, rosemary, sage and ½ the thyme. Cook, stirring, for 8 to 10 minutes or until mushroom is browned.

4. Add the stock and 1 ½ cups water. Bring to the boil. Return pork to dish. Cover. Transfer to oven. Bake for 1 hour 20 minutes or until pork is tender.

5. Meanwhile, cook barley following packet directions. Drain well. Cover to keep warm.

6. Uncover casserole dish. Bake for a further 15 minutes or until sauce thickens. Season with pepper. Combine parsley, lemon zest and remaining thyme in a bowl. Spoon pork mixture over barley. Sprinkle with gremolata and serve with broccolini.

Chicken With Tandoori Cauliflower And Herb Sauce

Ingredients

- 2 tablespoons vegetable oil

- 2 garlic cloves, crushed

- 2cm piece fresh ginger, finely grated

- 2 tablespoons chopped fresh coriander leaves

- 4 large chicken thigh cutlets, skin on

- 2 tablespoons tandoori paste

- 1 tablespoon finely grated lemon rind

- 1 tablespoon honey

- 1 large (1kg) cauliflower, cut into thick wedges

- 200g plain Greek-style yoghurt

- 2 teaspoons lemon juice

- ½ cup fresh coriander leaves

- ½ cup fresh flat-leaf parsley leaves

- 200g green beans, trimmed

- 80g baby spinach

- 2 tablespoons natural flaked almonds, toasted

- 1 lemon, cut into wedges

Preparation

1. Preheat oven to 220C/200C fan-forced. Line a large baking tray with baking paper.

2. Combine half the oil, garlic, ginger and chopped coriander in a bowl. Trim excess fat from chicken. Place chicken on prepared tray. Rub all over with oil mixture. Roast, skin-side up, for 15 minutes.

3. Combine remaining oil, curry paste, lemon rind and honey in a large bowl. Add cauliflower, rubbing with mixture to coat. Place on tray with chicken. Bake for a further 25 minutes or until cauliflower is golden and tender and chicken is cooked through.

4. Meanwhile, place yoghurt, lemon juice, ¼ cup coriander leaves and ¼ cup parsley in a small food processor. Process until smooth and combined.

5. Cook beans in a medium saucepan of boiling water for 1 minute or until just tender. Drain. Refresh under cold water. Drain well. Place beans, spinach, almonds and remaining coriander and parsley leaves in a bowl. Toss to combine.

6. Serve chicken and cauliflower with herb sauce, bean salad and lemon wedges.

Quinoa-crumbed veal schnitzel with shaved fennel and apple salad

Ingredients

- ½ cup rice flour
- 1/3 cup milk
- 1 egg
- 1 ½ cups quinoa flakes
- 2 tablespoons finely chopped fresh chives
- 2 teaspoons finely grated lemon rind
- 4 x 125g veal schnitzels (uncrumbed)
- 1 fennel, fronds reserved
- 2 small pink lady apples
- 2 cups watercress sprigs
- 2 tablespoons lemon juice
- 1 tablespoon extra virgin olive oil
- 1 teaspoon wholegrain mustard
- Vegetable oil, for shallow-frying

• Lemon wedges, to serve

Preparation

1. Place rice flour on a plate. Season with salt and pepper. Whisk milk and egg in a shallow bowl until combined. Combine quinoa, chives and lemon rind on a plate.

2. Toss 1 piece veal schnitzel in rice flour mixture, shaking off excess. Dip in egg mixture. Coat in quinoa mixture, pressing down firmly. Place on a tray. Repeat with remaining veal, rice flour, egg and quinoa mixtures. Refrigerate for 10 minutes.

3. Meanwhile, using a mandolin or sharp knife, thinly shave fennel. Halve and core apples. Cut into thin wedges. Combine fennel, reserved fennel fronds, apple and watercress in a medium bowl.

4. Whisk lemon juice, oil and mustard in a small bowl to combine. Season with salt and pepper. Add dressing to fennel mixture. Toss to combine.

5. Pour enough oil into a large frying pan to come 5mm up side of pan. Heat over medium-high heat. Cook schnitzels for 2 minutes each side or until just cooked through. Drain on paper towel. Serve schnitzels with fennel and apple salad and lemon wedges.

Roast chicken with spicy green butter

Ingredients

- 70g butter, chopped, at room temperature

- ¼ cup fresh coriander leaves, finely chopped

- 1 tablespoon finely chopped fresh green chilli

- 2 teaspoons finely grated fresh ginger

- 1 lime, rind finely grated, juiced

- 2 bunches baby carrots, trimmed, scrubbed

- 1 red onion, cut into wedges

- 2 teaspoons honey

- 4 (about 1kg) chicken supremes, French-trimmed

- 200g green beans, trimmed

Preparation

1. Preheat oven to 200°C/180°C fan forced. Line 2 baking trays with baking paper. Place the butter, coriander, chilli, ginger and lime rind in a bowl and use a wooden spoon to beat until combined.

2. Combine the carrot, onion, honey, 3 tsp of the butter mixture and 2 tablespoons lime juice in a bowl. Season. Place on 1 prepared tray. Roast on top oven shelf for 12 minutes.

3. Meanwhile, heat a large non-stick frying pan over medium-high heat. Spray the chicken with oil. Season.

Cook, skin-side down, for 4 minutes or until golden. Turn and cook for 3 minutes. Transfer to the second prepared tray. Top each piece of chicken with 1 teaspoon butter mixture.

4. Roast chicken on the lower oven shelf for 15-18 minutes or until cooked through. Keep warm.

5. Increase oven to 220°C/200°C fan forced. Add beans to the vegie tray. Toss to coat in pan juices. Roast for a further 6-8 minutes or until beans are tender-crisp. Serve chicken with the vegies. Top with remaining butter.

Cheesy Apple Toastie

Ingredients

• 1 slice Swiss cheese such as Edam, Gouda or Emmental

• 4 thin slices of red apple

• 2 slices white bread (or gluten free bread)

• Olive oil spray

Preparation

1. Preheat the sandwich maker

2. Spray both sides of both piece of bread lightly

3. Make the sandwich by placing the apple slices on the bottom piece of bread and cheese on top

4. Add the top piece of bread

5. Close the sandwich maker and toast until golden.

Roasted Apple and Veggies

Ingredients

• 2 parsnips (peeled and sliced thickly length ways)

• 1 large carrot (peeled and sliced thickly length ways)

• 2 large red skinned potatoes (peeled and cut into chunks)

• 2 large red apples (cored and sliced into four)

• 4 sprigs of Thyme* (leaves separated from the twig)

• 4 tbsp extra virgin olive oil

• Cracked salt and pepper to taste

Preparation

1. Heat oven to 180C for 20 minutes

2. Place all ingredients in a large bowl and coat with olive oil and ensure the vegetables are coated with the oil and thyme leaves (or powder)

3. Place contents on baking paper in a baking tray and cook for 40-50 minutes until th

4. Enjoy with your favourite winter meals.

Pink Lady Smoothie

Ingredients

- 350 ml water or milk of your choice

- 1 large scoop of whey or pea protein vanilla flavoured

- 1 large banana (peeled)

- 1 Pink Lady apple (finely chopped for blending)

- 1 tbsp minute oats

- ½ cup ice if you prefer a cold drink

Preparation

1. Soak minute oats in water for 10 minutes before blending

2. Blend water/milk with chia seeds, protein powder, banana, and chopped apple in a blender until all ingredients are smooth

3. Serve with a sprig of mint.

Apple Sausage Pasta

Ingredients

- 450 grams chicken sausages (or veggie sausages)

- 1 Green apple (peeled, cored and chopped into chunks)

- ½ large brown onion (finely diced)

- 2 tsp garlic powder

- 500 ml low salt chicken/vegetable stock

- 400 ml pasata

- 300 grams pasta

- 1 cup shredded cheddar cheese

- 1 tbsp extra-virgin olive oil

- Salt and pepper to taste

Preparation

1. In a large frying pan (must have a lid) add the olive oil and heat to medium heat.

2. Cook the onions, garlic and sausages for about 10 minutes until golden.

3. Let the sausages cool and slice them thinly and add back to the pan and heat again to medium with the chopped apple until apple is soft.

4. Add the stock and pasata, stirring to ensure the mixture is blended through, add salt and pepper to taste and bring to a boil.

5. Add the pasta and the lid and cook until the pasta is cooked, stirring regularly to ensure the pasta does not stick at the bottom of the pan.

6. Stir until the liquid has evaporated, stir cheese through at the last minute.

7. Serve with a side of steamed vegetables.